THE

IVF DIET

COOKBOOK

SARAH JACK

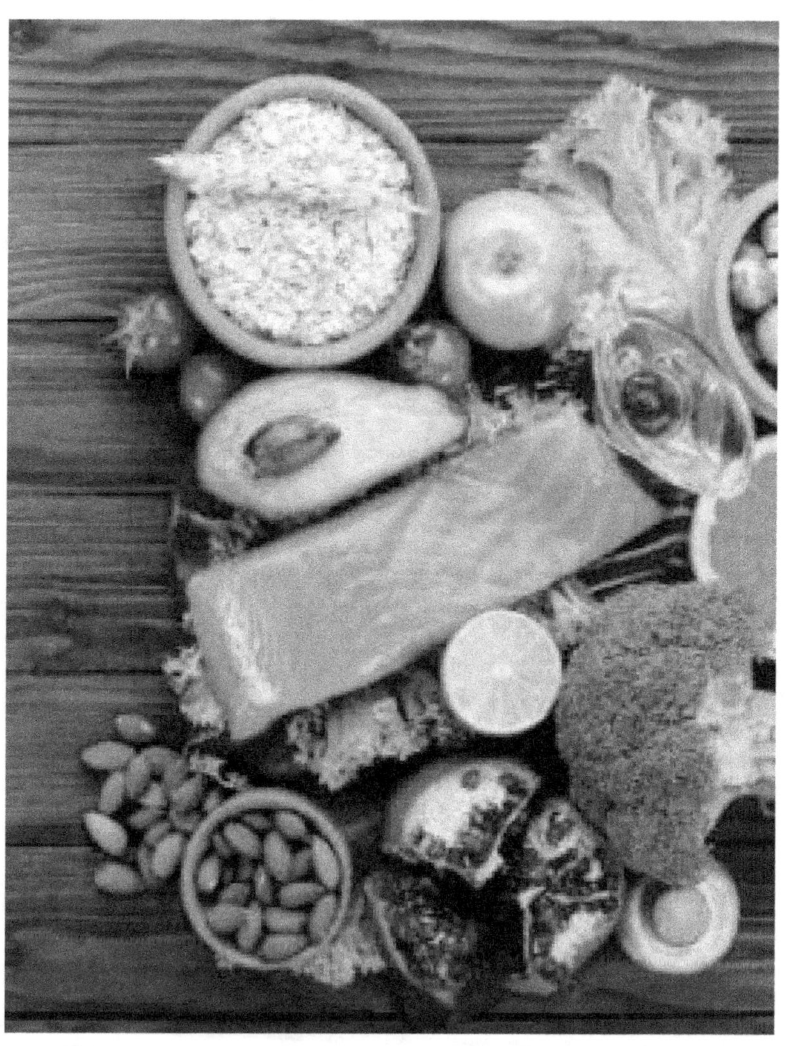

COPYRIGHT

TABLE OF CONTENTS

INTRODUCTION

IVF

In Vitro Fertilization (IVF) has revolutionized the field of reproductive medicine, offering hope to individuals and couples facing challenges in conceiving naturally. Since the birth of the first IVF baby, Louise Brown, in 1978, this assisted reproductive technology (ART) has evolved significantly, becoming a widely utilized and successful method for achieving pregnancy. In this comprehensive overview, we will delve into the various aspects of IVF, including the process, success rates, ethical considerations, and the emotional journey associated with fertility treatments.

- **Understanding IVF: The Process**

Ovulation Induction:

The IVF process typically begins with ovulation induction. Fertility medications are administered to stimulate the ovaries to produce multiple eggs. Monitoring through blood tests and ultrasounds is conducted to track follicle development. This step aims to maximize the number of mature eggs retrieved during the next phase.

Egg Retrieval:

Once the follicles reach the desired size, a minor surgical procedure known as egg retrieval is performed. This is usually done under sedation. A thin needle is guided through the vaginal wall to the ovaries, and the eggs are aspirated from the follicles. The retrieved eggs are then placed in a special culture medium and transferred to the laboratory for fertilization.

Sperm Collection and Fertilization:

Sperm is collected from the male partner or a sperm donor. In the laboratory, the eggs and sperm are combined to facilitate fertilization. This can be achieved through conventional insemination, where sperm is added to the eggs, or through intracytoplasmic sperm injection (ICSI), where a single sperm is directly injected into an egg. The fertilized eggs, now called embryos, are cultured for several days.

Embryo Transfer:

After a few days of monitoring, the healthiest embryos are selected for transfer. The number of embryos transferred is determined based on various factors, including the woman's age and the quality of the embryos. The embryo transfer is a relatively simple procedure where the selected embryos are placed into the woman's uterus using a thin catheter. Any remaining high-quality embryos may be cryopreserved for future use.

Luteal Phase Support:

To support the potential implantation of the embryos, hormonal medications such as progesterone are administered during the luteal phase. These medications help prepare the uterine lining for embryo implantation and support early pregnancy.

- **Success Rates and Factors Affecting IVF Outcomes**

IVF success rates vary based on several factors, including the age of the woman, the cause of infertility, and the quality of the embryos. Generally, younger women tend to have higher success rates because they often produce healthier eggs. The overall success rates have improved over the years due to advancements in technology, laboratory techniques, and better understanding of reproductive physiology.

Factors influencing IVF success include:

Age:

Female age is a crucial determinant of success. As women age, the quality and quantity of their eggs decline, affecting the chances of successful fertilization and implantation.

Embryo Quality:

High-quality embryos have a higher chance of successful implantation. Advances in embryo selection techniques, such as preimplantation genetic testing (PGT), help identify chromosomally normal embryos, improving the likelihood of a healthy pregnancy.

Cause of Infertility:

The underlying cause of infertility can impact IVF success. Conditions such as tubal factor infertility, male factor infertility, or unexplained infertility may have different success rates.

Number of Embryos Transferred:

While transferring multiple embryos may increase the chances of pregnancy, it also raises the risk of multiple pregnancies, which come with their own set of challenges and potential complications.

Lifestyle Factors:

Factors such as body weight, smoking, and overall health can influence IVF success. Maintaining a healthy lifestyle before and during treatment is advisable.

- **Ethical Considerations in IVF**

IVF has brought about profound ethical considerations, prompting ongoing discussions and debates. Some of the key ethical considerations include:

Selective Reduction:

In cases where multiple embryos implant, there is a risk of a high-order multiple pregnancy (triplets or more). Selective reduction, the process of reducing the number of implanted embryos to a manageable number, raises ethical questions about the value of each individual life.

Cryopreservation and Disposition of Unused Embryos:

Couples often face decisions about what to do with unused embryos. Options include cryopreservation for future use, donation to others, research donation, or discarding. These choices can be emotionally challenging and involve complex ethical considerations.

Preimplantation Genetic Testing (PGT):

PGT is used to identify chromosomal abnormalities in embryos before implantation. While it can help prevent the transfer of embryos with genetic disorders, it also raises ethical concerns about the selection of desirable traits and potential misuse of the technology.

Access and Affordability:

The cost of IVF and its accessibility raise ethical questions about who has access to these treatments. Financial barriers can limit the ability of some individuals and couples to pursue IVF, leading to disparities in access to reproductive healthcare.

- **Emotional Aspects of IVF**

The journey through IVF is emotionally charged, with both highs and lows. The emotional aspects of IVF include:

Hope and Anticipation:

The decision to undergo IVF is often fueled by a strong desire for parenthood. Couples embark on the process with hope and anticipation, eagerly awaiting positive results.

Stress and Anxiety:

The IVF process, with its numerous steps and uncertainties, can be stressful. The fear of failure and the financial investment can contribute to heightened anxiety levels.

Disappointment and Grief:

IVF outcomes are not guaranteed, and unsuccessful cycles can be emotionally challenging. Couples may experience grief, disappointment, and a sense of loss.

Joy and Relief:

On the flip side, successful IVF cycles bring immense joy and relief. The positive pregnancy test and the realization of becoming parents can be a transformative and joyous moment.

Navigating Relationships:

The emotional toll of IVF can impact relationships. Open communication, support, and shared decision-making are essential for couples navigating the complexities of fertility treatments.

- **Future Directions and Innovations in IVF**

As technology and research continue to advance, the field of IVF is witnessing ongoing innovations. Some areas of focus include:

Innovations in Embryo Culture:

Improving the conditions in which embryos are cultured can enhance their development, potentially leading to higher success rates.

Advancements in Genetic Testing:

Ongoing developments in genetic testing techniques aim to refine the selection of embryos with the highest chances of success while minimizing ethical concerns.

Fertility Preservation:

IVF is increasingly being used for fertility preservation, allowing individuals to freeze their eggs or embryos for later use, especially important for those facing medical treatments that may impact fertility.

Precision Medicine in Reproductive Health:

Personalized treatment approaches, based on individual genetic and physiological characteristics, may become more prevalent, optimizing outcomes for each patient.

Artificial Intelligence in IVF:

The integration of artificial intelligence (AI) in analyzing data from IVF cycles may contribute to more accurate predictions of success and personalized treatment plans.

- **Conclusion**

In Vitro Fertilization has transformed the landscape of reproductive medicine, providing a lifeline to individuals and couples grappling with infertility. While the emotional and ethical considerations associated with IVF are complex, the continuous advancements in technology offer hope for improved success rates and more personalized treatment approaches. As research and innovation progress, the future of IVF holds the promise of expanding access, reducing ethical dilemmas, and increasing the likelihood of successful outcomes for those on the journey to parenthood. The decision to pursue IVF is deeply personal, and individuals and couples are encouraged to seek support, guidance, and information to make informed choices aligned with their values and aspirations.

WHAT IS IVF DIET?

There isn't a certain "IVF diet" that is always suggested for people undergoing in vitro fertilization (IVF). But when preparing for IVF or any reproductive therapy, eating a balanced, healthy diet can be helpful. A healthy diet can support general well-being, promote optimal reproductive function, and increase the likelihood of a successful pregnancy. For those undergoing IVF, the following dietary recommendations and considerations are provided:

- Maintain a balanced diet by consuming a range of foods from all dietary groups, such as fruits, vegetables, whole grains, lean proteins, and dairy or dairy substitutes. This guarantees that you receive a variety of crucial nutrients.

- Including foods high in folate, such as leafy greens, lentils, and fortified cereals, is a good idea because folate is necessary for fetal development. A prenatal vitamin containing folic acid is also advised by many medical professionals to be taken before and throughout pregnancy.

- Omega-3 Fatty Acids: Omega-3 fatty acids can enhance reproductive health and may help reduce inflammation. They are present in fatty fish (such as salmon), flaxseeds, and walnuts.

- Limit Processed Meals: Eat less highly processed and sugary meals because they may have a detrimental impact on fertility as well as general health.

- Maintain a Healthy Weight: It's crucial for fertility to reach and keep a healthy weight. Hormone levels and menstrual regularity might be affected by being underweight or overweight. For advice on how to reach a healthy weight, speak with a healthcare professional.

- Maintain Proper Hydration: Proper hydration is essential. To maintain good general health and to support your body's functions, drink lots of water.

- Limiting caffeine and alcohol use during reproductive treatments, including IVF, is advised by certain healthcare professionals. It is best to adhere to the precise suggestions made in this regard by your healthcare provider.

- Supplements: Your doctor may suggest certain supplements, like coenzyme Q10, vitamin D, or others, in addition to a balanced diet to boost fertility. Before beginning any new supplements, always get medical advice.

- Stress reduction is crucial throughout IVF and other fertility therapies. Include stress-reduction practices into your daily routine, such as mindfulness, meditation, yoga, or counseling.

- Consult a Registered Dietitian or Nutritionist: If you have certain dietary issues or conditions that may affect fertility, think about visiting with one of these professionals. They can offer you individualized advice and suggestions that are catered to your needs.

Keep in mind that every person has unique nutritional requirements and fertility considerations. Therefore, it's critical to collaborate closely with your healthcare team, which may include a dietician and a fertility specialist, to create a strategy that is tailored to your unique needs and objectives. A balanced diet and a healthy lifestyle that includes regular exercise and enough sleep can also help with general wellbeing during the IVF process.

BENEFITS OF IVF DIET

There isn't a particular "IVF diet" with special advantages. However, when undergoing in vitro fertilization (IVF) or other reproductive therapy, keeping a healthy and balanced diet might offer various general benefits, including:

- Overall Health: A balanced diet supports your overall health, including your reproductive system. Nutrient-rich foods provide essential vitamins and mincrals that are necessary for various bodily functions, including hormone regulation and egg/sperm quality.

- A healthy diet helps to manage hormone levels, which is essential for a successful IVF cycle. In the growth and development of eggs and sperm, hormones are crucial.

- Weight management: Eating a healthy weight is possible with the help of a balanced diet. Both being underweight and being overweight can harm fertility. Keeping a healthy weight can increase the likelihood that an IVF cycle will be successful.

- Reduced Inflammation: Some meals, such as those high in omega-3 fatty acids (such fatty fish and flaxseeds), can have anti-inflammatory effects. By improving the conditions for implantation and pregnancy, decreased inflammation can help fertility.

- Antioxidants and critical nutrients found in nutrient-dense diets can help to improve the quality of eggs and sperm, which may increase the possibility of an IVF cycle being successful.

- Folate and the Prevention of Neural Tube malformations: In order to protect the developing baby against neural tube malformations, foliate-rich meals and folic acid supplements are crucial. Increasing the amount of folate a woman consumes is frequently advised, including during IVF.

- Reduced Risk of Complications: Gestational diabetes and preeclampsia are two conditions that can be lessened in risk by following a balanced diet. The ultimate objective is a fruitful IVF cycle followed by a healthy pregnancy.

- Optimized Energy Levels: Emotionally and physically taxing as IVF can be, proper nutrition can improve overall wellbeing by helping to sustain energy levels.

- Eating healthfully can help improve mental well-being and stress management. During fertility treatments, it's critical to reduce stress because it can harm fertility.

- Support for Men's Fertility: Men undergoing IVF should maintain a healthy diet as well. Foods high in nutrients can enhance the quality and mobility of sperm.

It's crucial to remember that while a good diet may provide these possible benefits, a successful IVF cycle may not necessarily result from it. Age, underlying medical issues, the precise reason of infertility, and a patient's response to treatment are just a few variables that can affect the results of IVF.

It's crucial to speak with a healthcare professional or a fertility specialist before beginning any supplements or making any dietary changes. Based on your unique circumstances and medical background, they can offer advice that are tailored to you. A licensed dietitian or nutritionist can also assist in developing a diet plan that supports your fertility objectives.

IMPORTANCE OF WATER INTAKE DURING IVF

The article emphasizes the crucial role of water intake in the success of In Vitro Fertilization (IVF). It highlights various aspects of the fertility process that are influenced by adequate hydration:

- **Optimal Follicular Development:**

Adequate water intake is essential for the production of healthy and mature eggs during the ovarian stimulation phase of IVF. Water serves as a medium for transporting nutrients and hormones to the ovaries, supporting optimal follicular development.

- **Cervical Mucus Quality and Sperm Transport:**

Hydration contributes to the production of healthy cervical mucus, which is vital for facilitating sperm motility and transport toward the egg. Insufficient water intake may result in less fertile cervical mucus, affecting the chances of successful fertilization.

- **Uterine Environment and Implantation Success:**

A well-hydrated body supports the overall health of the uterine lining, a critical factor in the successful implantation of embryos. Maintaining optimal hydration levels ensures the uterine lining remains receptive, increasing the likelihood of successful embryo implantation.

- **Mitigating Ovarian Hyperstimulation Syndrome (OHSS):**

Proper hydration plays a crucial role in reducing the risk and severity of OHSS, a potential complication of ovarian stimulation in IVF. Well-hydrated individuals are better equipped to handle the fluid imbalances associated with this syndrome.

- **Blood Circulation and Nutrient Transport:**

Hydration is closely linked to optimal blood circulation, crucial for transporting nutrients and hormones to the reproductive organs. Proper hydration ensures a consistent supply of essential substances to the ovaries and uterus, supporting the development of healthy eggs and a receptive uterine lining.

- **Stress Reduction and Hormonal Balance:**

Hydration contributes to stress reduction and hormonal balance, essential for reproductive health. Maintaining adequate water intake helps regulate stress hormones, fostering emotional well-being during the emotionally charged IVF journey.

- **Post-Transfer Recovery:**

Proper hydration remains important after the embryo transfer. While rest is recommended, adequate hydration supports the body's recovery, contributing to overall well-being and potentially reducing the risk of complications.

In conclusion, the article emphasizes that water intake is a fundamental aspect of the IVF journey, influencing various physiological processes crucial for successful fertility treatment. Couples undergoing IVF are encouraged to recognize the importance of staying hydrated as a proactive and empowering element in their quest to build a family through assisted reproductive technologies. Adequate hydration is portrayed as a silent ally, nourishing the path to conception with each refreshing sip.

IVF DIET RECIPES

Vegetable Omelette

Ingredients:

- Three big eggs

- Diced bell peppers, 1/4 cup

- Diced tomatoes, 1/4 cup

- 4 cups of spinach leaves

- Sliced mushrooms, 1/4 cup

- Pepper and salt as desired

- Cooking spray or olive oil for the pan

Instructions:

- In a bowl, whisk the eggs and season with salt and pepper.

- Heat a non-stick skillet over medium heat and lightly coat it with cooking spray or olive oil.

- Pour the whisked eggs into the skillet.

- Sprinkle the spinach, mushrooms, tomatoes, bell peppers, and spinach equally over one half of the omelette.

- When the eggs are set but still slightly runny on top, carefully fold the other half over the veggies.

- Cook for a few more minutes until the omelette is fully cooked.

- Slide it onto a plate, and enjoy.

Avocado and Spinach Smoothie

Ingredients:

- 1 ripe avocado

- Spinach leaves, 1 cup

- Half a banana

- A half-cup of unsweetened almond milk (or another type of milk)

- 1 tablespoon of maple syrup or honey

- Ice cubes, if desired

Instructions:

- In a blender, mix all the ingredients until they are smooth and creamy.

- Add ice cubes if you want a colder smoothie.

Berry and Nut Parfait

Ingredients:

- Greek yogurt (full-fat or low-fat)

- Mixed berries (e.g., strawberries, blueberries, raspberries)

- Chopped nuts (e.g., almonds, walnuts)

- Honey or maple syrup

Instructions:

- Layer Greek yogurt, a variety of berries, and chopped almonds in a glass or bowl.

- For sweetness, drizzle with honey or maple syrup.

Broccoli and White Bean Soup

Ingredients:

- 2 cups broccoli florets

- 1 can (15 oz) white beans, drained and rinsed

- 1 onion, chopped

- 2 minced garlic cloves

- 4 cups low-sodium vegetable broth

- One tablespoon of dried thyme

- Pepper and salt as desired

Instructions:

- Olive oil should be used to sauté chopped onion and minced garlic until they are tender.

- Add white beans, dried thyme, salt, and pepper along with the broccoli florets and vegetable broth.

- Bring to a boil, then lower the heat and simmer the broccoli for 15 to 20 minutes, or until it is soft.

- Use an immersion blender to puree the soup until smooth. Alternatively, carefully transfer the soup to a blender in batches, blend, and return it to the pot.

- Before serving, adjust the seasoning as necessary.

Caprese Salad

Ingredients:

- Sliced fresh tomatoes

- Sliced fresh mozzarella cheese

- Fresh leaves of basil

- Olive oil extra virgin

- Balsamic glaze, if desired

- Pepper and salt as desired

Instructions:

- On a serving platter, alternately arrange tomato and mozzarella slices.

- Place some fresh basil between the pieces.

- Balsamic glaze (if using) and extra-virgin olive oil should be drizzled over top.

- Add salt and pepper to taste.

- Serve as a light and refreshing salad.

Mediterranean Tuna Salad

Ingredients:

- Canned tuna in water, drained

- Cherry tomatoes, halved

- Cucumber, diced

- Kalamata olives, pitted and halved

- Red onion, thinly sliced

- Feta cheese crumbles (optional)

- Fresh parsley, chopped

- Extra-virgin olive oil

- Lemon juice

- Pepper and salt as desired

Instructions:

- Canned tuna, cherry tomatoes, chopped cucumber, Kalamata olives, thinly sliced red onion, and crumbled feta cheese (if using) should all be combined in a bowl.

- Lemon juice and extra virgin olive oil should be drizzled on.

- Add salt and pepper to taste.

- Prior to serving, garnish with freshly chopped parsley.

Baked Cod with Lemon and Dill

Ingredients:

- 4 fillets of cod

- One lemon's juice and zest

- Freshly sliced dill

- 2 minced garlic cloves

- Olive oil, two tablespoons

- Pepper and salt as desired

Instructions:

- Set the oven's temperature to 375°F (190°C).

- In a bowl, mix lemon zest, lemon juice, chopped fresh dill, minced garlic, olive oil, salt, and pepper.

- Cod fillets should be placed on a baking pan covered with parchment paper.

- Pour the lemon-dill mixture over the cod.

- Bake the fish for 15 to 20 minutes, or until it flakes easily with a fork.

Chocolate Avocado Mousse

Ingredients:

- Two ripe avocados

- Unsweetened cocoa powder, 1/4 cup

- 1/4 cup maple syrup or honey

- Vanilla extract, 1 teaspoon

- A pinch of salt

- Fresh berries for topping (optional)

- Instructions:

- Scoop the flesh of the avocados into a blender or food processor.

- Add vanilla essence, honey or maple syrup, cocoa powder, and a dash of salt.

- Blend till creamy and smooth.

- Divide the mousse into serving dishes and refrigerate for at least 30 minutes before serving.

- Fresh berries can optionally be sprinkled on top to enhance taste and texture.

Baked Vegetable Frittata

Ingredients:

- 8 large eggs

- 1 cup mixed vegetables (e.g., bell peppers, spinach, mushrooms), chopped

- 1/2 cup grated cheese (e.g., cheddar, mozzarella)

- 1/4 cup milk (dairy or non-dairy)

- A half-teaspoon of dried oregano

- Pepper and salt as desired

- Cooking spray or olive oil for the pan

Instructions:

- Set the oven's temperature to 350°F (175°C).

- Combine the eggs, milk, dried oregano, salt, and pepper in a bowl.

- Heat an oven-safe skillet over medium heat and coat it with cooking spray or olive oil.

- In the skillet, add the chopped vegetables and cook for a few minutes, or until they start to soften.

- Pour the egg mixture over the vegetables and sprinkle grated cheese evenly.

- Transfer the skillet to the preheated oven and bake for about 15-20 minutes, or until the frittata is set and slightly golden.

- Slice, then dish.

Teriyaki Salmon with Boccoli

Ingredients:

- 2 fillets of salmon

- Broccoli florets in a cup

- Low-sodium teriyaki sauce, 1/4 cup

- 1 teaspoon of honey

- Low-sodium soy sauce, 1 tbsp

- 1 minced garlic clove

- A teaspoon of freshly grated ginger

- Sesame seeds for garnish (optional)

- Cooked brown rice for serving

Instructions:

- Set the oven's temperature to 375°F (190°C).

- Teriyaki sauce, honey, low-sodium soy sauce, minced garlic, and grated ginger should all be combined in a bowl.

- On a baking sheet, arrange the broccoli and salmon fillets.

- Salmon and broccoli are covered in a spray of the teriyaki sauce.

- Bake for 15 to 20 minutes, or until the broccoli is soft and the salmon flakes easily with a fork.

- If preferred, top with sesame seeds and serve with cooked brown rice.

Quinoa and Chickpea Stuffed Bell Peppers

Ingredients:

- 4 bell peppers, any color

- 1 cup cooked quinoa

- 1 can (15 oz) washed and drained chickpeas

- Diced tomatoes, 1 cup

- 1 teaspoon of cumin, ground

- Paprika, half a teaspoon

- Pepper and salt as desired

- Fresh cilantro leaves for garnish (optional)

Instructions:

- Set the oven's temperature to 375°F (190°C).

- Remove the bell peppers' tops, then scoop out the seeds and membranes.

- Cooked quinoa, chickpeas, diced tomatoes, cumin, paprika, salt, and pepper should all be combined in a bowl.

- Put the quinoa mixture inside the bell peppers.

- The filled peppers should be placed on a baking dish and covered with foil.

- Bake the peppers for 25 to 30 minutes, or until they are soft.

- Before serving, you could add some fresh cilantro as a garnish.

Greek Tzatziki Sauce

Ingredients:

- 1 cup Greek yogurt (full-fat or low-fat)

- 1 cucumber, grated and squeezed to remove excess moisture

- 2 minced garlic cloves

- 1 tablespoon finely sliced fresh dill

- 1 tablespoon minced fresh mint

- Extra virgin olive oil, 1 tablespoon

- Juice of 1/2 lemon

- Pepper and salt as desired

Instructions:

- Greek yogurt, grated cucumber, minced garlic, fresh dill and mint cut, olive oil, lemon juice, salt, and pepper are all combined in a basin.

- Mix thoroughly.

- Refrigerate for at least 30 minutes before serving.

- Serve as a dip with fresh vegetables or as a sauce for grilled chicken or fish.

Moroccan Chickpea Stew

Ingredients:

- 2 cans of chickpeas (15 oz each), drained and rinsed

- One chopped onion

- 2 minced garlic cloves

- 1 can of diced tomatoes (14 oz).

- 1 cup low-sodium vegetable broth

- 1 teaspoon of cumin, ground

- 1 teaspoon of coriander, ground

- 1/2 teaspoon cinnamon powder

- Pepper and salt as desired

- Fresh cilantro leaves can be used as a garnish.

Instructions:

- Olive oil should be used to cook chopped onions and minced garlic until they are tender.

- Add salt, pepper, ground cinnamon, ground coriander, and ground cumin. Stir for a minute.

- Add the veggie broth, diced tomatoes, and chickpeas.

- Bring to a boil before lowering the heat, covering the pot, and simmering for 20 to 25 minutes.

- If preferred, garnish the food with fresh cilantro leaves before serving.

Thai-Inspired Peanut Chicken

Ingredients:

- 2 boneless, skinless chicken breasts, cut into strips

- 1/2 cup unsweetened peanut butter

- Low-sodium soy sauce, two tablespoons

- 1 tablespoon of maple syrup or honey

- 1 lime's juice

- 2 minced garlic cloves

- A teaspoon of freshly grated ginger

- Flakes of red pepper, crushed (optional)

- Chopped cilantro for garnish

- Cooked brown rice for serving

Instructions:

- Peanut butter, low-sodium soy sauce, honey or maple syrup, lime juice, ginger, garlic, and crushed red pepper flakes (if using) should all be combined in a bowl.

- Heat a skillet over medium-high heat and lightly coat it with cooking spray or olive oil.

- Cook the chicken strips after being added until they are thoroughly done.

- Pour the peanut sauce over the cooked chicken and stir to coat.

- Serve with chopped cilantro as a garnish over cooked brown rice.

Roasted Brussels Sprouts with Balsamic Glaze

Ingredients:

- Brussels sprouts, trimmed and halved

- Olive oil, two tablespoons

- Pepper and salt as desired

- Balsamic glaze

Instructions:

- Set the oven's temperature to 400°F (200°C).

- Toss halved Brussels sprouts with olive oil, salt, and pepper.

- On a baking sheet, spread them out.

- Roast for 25 to 30 minutes in a preheated oven, or until fork-tender and slightly browned.

- Drizzle with balsamic glaze before serving.

Cilantro Lime Shrimp Tacos

Ingredients:

- 1 pound of peeled and deveined big shrimp

- One lime's juice and zest

- 2 minced garlic cloves

- 2 teaspoons chopped fresh cilantro

- Olive oil, 1 tbsp

- Pepper and salt as desired

- Corn or whole-grain tortillas

- Sliced avocado, diced tomatoes, shredded lettuce for toppings

Instructions:

- Olive oil, salt, pepper, minced garlic, cilantro, and lime zest should all be combined in a bowl.

- Add the shrimp to the bowl and toss to coat. Give it around 15 minutes to marinate.

- Heat a skillet over medium-high heat and cook the shrimp for about 2-3 minutes per side or until they turn pink and opaque.

- In a microwave or a dry skillet, reheat the tortillas.

- Fill the tortillas with cooked shrimp and top with sliced avocado, diced tomatoes, and shredded lettuce.

Asparagus and Parmesan Risotto

Ingredients:

- Arborio rice, 1 cup

- 2 cups low-sodium vegetable broth

- 1 bunch of trimmed and cubed bite-sized asparagus

- Grated Parmesan cheese, half a cup

- 2 tablespoons butter (or olive oil for a dairy-free option)

- Pepper and salt as desired

- For garnish, use fresh parsley.

Instructions:

- Butter (or olive oil) and Arborio rice should be sautéed over medium heat until the rice is lightly browned.

- Add a ladleful of vegetable broth and stir until absorbed by the rice.

- One ladle at a time, add broth as previously, stirring frequently and letting it absorb before adding more.

- About halfway through cooking (after about 10-12 minutes), add the asparagus pieces to the risotto.

- Continue adding broth and stirring until the rice and asparagus are cooked to your desired level of tenderness (usually around 18-20 minutes).

- Stir in grated Parmesan cheese and season with salt and pepper.

- If preferred, garnish the food with fresh parsley before serving.

Roasted Red Pepper Hummus

Ingredients:

- 1 can (15 oz) chickpeas, drained and rinsed

- 2 roasted red peppers (from a jar or homemade), drained

- 2 tablespoons tahini

- Juice of 1 lemon

- 2 cloves garlic, minced

- 1/2 teaspoon ground cumin

- Salt and pepper to taste

- Extra-virgin olive oil for drizzling

- Paprika and fresh parsley for garnish (optional)

- Pita bread or fresh vegetables for dipping

Instructions:

- Add chickpeas, roasted red peppers, tahini, lemon juice, minced garlic, ground cumin, salt, and pepper to a food processor.

- Process until smooth and creamy, scraping down the sides as needed

- Put the hummus in a bowl for serving.

- Sprinkle with paprika and fresh parsley, if preferred, and drizzle with extra-virgin olive oil.

- Serve with fresh vegetables or pita bread for dipping.

Honey Mustard Baked Salmon

Ingredients:

- 4 fillets of salmon

- Dijon mustard, two tablespoons

- Honey, two tablespoons

- 1 minced garlic clove

- One tablespoon of dried thyme

- Pepper and salt as desired

- Lemon wedges for serving

Instructions:

- Set the oven's temperature to 375°F (190°C).

- Dijon mustard, honey, minced garlic, dried thyme, salt, and pepper should all be combined in a bowl.

- Salmon fillets should be put on a baking pan covered with parchment paper.

- Brush the honey mustard mixture over the salmon.

- Salmon should easily flake with a fork after baking for 15 to 20 minutes.

- Lemon wedges can be added to the dish for flavor.

Teriyaki Tofu Stir-Fry

Ingredients:

- Cubed, firm tofu

- Mixed vegetables (e.g., broccoli, bell peppers, snap peas), sliced

- Low-sodium teriyaki sauce, 1/4 cup

- Olive oil, two tablespoons

- Sesame seeds for garnish (optional)

- Cooked brown rice for serving

Instructions:

- Olive oil should be heated over medium-high heat in a skillet.

- Cubed tofu should be added and cooked until it is just beginning to color.

- Remove tofu from the skillet and set aside.

- Sliced mixed veggies should be stir-fried in the same skillet until crisp-tender.

- Return the tofu to the skillet and add low-sodium teriyaki sauce.

- Cook for an additional 2-3 minutes, allowing the sauce to coat the tofu and vegetables.

- Serve with sesame seeds as a topping over cooked brown rice.

Baked Sweet Potato Fries

Ingredients:

- Sweet potatoes, cut into fries

- Olive oil

- Paprika

- Garlic powder

- Salt and pepper to taste

Instructions:

- Set the oven's temperature to 425°F (220°C).

- Olive oil, paprika, garlic powder, salt, and pepper are added to sweet potato fries.

- Spread them out on a baking sheet in a single layer.

- For 20 to 25 minutes, or until the fries are crispy and golden, bake in the preheated oven.

Butternut Squash and Apple Soup

Ingredients:

- 1 butternut squash, peeled, seeded, and diced

- 2 apples, peeled, cored, and diced

- One sliced onion

- 2 minced garlic cloves

- 4 cups low-sodium vegetable broth

- 1 teaspoon of cinnamon powder

- 1/2 teaspoon of nutmeg, ground

- Pepper and salt as desired

- Olive oil

- Greek yogurt or coconut cream can be used as a garnish.

Instructions:

- Olive oil is heated over medium heat in a big pot. Add the minced garlic and onion, and cook until they are softened.

- Add diced butternut squash and apples to the pot and cook for a few minutes.

- Pour in vegetable broth and add ground cinnamon and ground nutmeg.

- Bring to a boil, then reduce heat, cover, and simmer for about 20-25 minutes or until the squash and apples are tender.

- Use an immersion blender or regular blender to puree the soup until smooth.

- Add salt and pepper to taste.

- If preferred, top with Greek yogurt or coconut cream when serving.

Mediterranean Stuffed Bell Peppers

Ingredients:

- 4 bell peppers, any color

- 1 cup cooked quinoa

- 1 can (15 oz) chickpeas, drained and rinsed

- Cherry tomatoes, halved

- Kalamata olives, pitted and halved

- Feta cheese crumbles

- Fresh parsley, chopped

- Extra-virgin olive oil

- Lemon juice

- Pepper and salt as desired

Instructions:

- Set the oven's temperature to 375°F (190°C).

- Remove the bell peppers' tops, then scoop out the seeds and membranes.

- Cooked quinoa, chickpeas, cherry tomatoes, Kalamata olives, and fresh parsley should all be combined in a big bowl.

- Sprinkle with feta cheese crumbles.

- Lemon juice and extra virgin olive oil should be drizzled on.

- Season with salt and pepper and toss to combine.

- Stuff the mixture into the bell peppers.

- The filled peppers should be placed on a baking dish and covered with foil.

- Bake the peppers for 25 to 30 minutes, or until they are soft.

- Before serving, you could add more fresh parsley as a garnish.

Greek-Style Baked Chicken Breasts

Ingredients:

- 4 boneless, skinless chicken breasts

- Greek seasoning blend (or a mix of dried oregano, basil, thyme, and garlic powder)

- Lemon juice

- Olive oil

- Salt and pepper to taste

- Feta cheese crumbles

- Sliced Kalamata olives

- Sliced cherry tomatoes

- Fresh parsley for garnish (optional)

Instructions:

- Set the oven's temperature to 375°F (190°C).

- Season chicken breasts with Greek seasoning blend, lemon juice, olive oil, salt, and pepper.

- In a baking dish, put the chicken breasts that have been spiced.

- Add feta cheese crumbles, Kalamata olive slices, and cherry tomato slices as garnish.

- Cook the chicken thoroughly in the preheated oven for around 25 to 30 minutes.

- If preferred, garnish the food with fresh parsley before serving.

Avocado and Tomato Salsa

Ingredients:

- Avocado, diced

- Tomatoes, diced

- Red onion, finely chopped

- Fresh cilantro, chopped

- Lime juice

- Pepper and salt as desired

- Crackers or tortilla chips for dipping

Instructions:

- Diced avocado, diced tomatoes, red onion, and fresh cilantro should all be combined in a bowl.

- Add lime juice as a drizzle.

- Add salt and pepper to taste.

- Gently blend by tossing.

- For a tasty snack or appetizer, serve with tortilla chips or crackers.

THANKS FOR

READING

THIS BOOK.